Jaime Harmer
PO Box 400448
Hesperia, CA 92340

jaimeharmer.com

First Edition
ISBN-13: 978-1974224913   ISBN-10: 1974224910

Cover silhouette image Created by Freepik
Cover Design by Sam & Jaime Harmer
Proofreading by Brittany Walker

<u>Works Cited</u>

CDC. "Vaccines and Preventable Diseases." Centers for Disease Control and Prevention. Centers for Disease Control and Prevention, 15 Dec. 2016. Web.

CDC. "What Should I Know About Screening?" Centers for Disease Control and Prevention. Centers for Disease Control and Prevention, 29 Mar. 2016. Web. 24 Aug. 2017.

Health, Amita. "Medical Disclaimer." Amita Health. Amita Health, n.d. Web. 13 Sept. 2017.

MD, Web. "Why Am I Bleeding After Menopause?" WebMD. WebMD, knwn. Web. 24 Aug. 2017.

Streicher, Lauren, MD. "Over 50: Bleeding After Menopause? Don't Go With That Flow!" Blog post. The Dr. Oz Show. N.p., 2011. Web. 24 Aug. 2017.

TABLE OF CONTENTS

DEDICATION

I dedicate this book to my husband, Sam,
who without his not so gentle persuasion,
I probably would never have written this.
Thank You

SO, WHAT'S THIS BOOK ALL ABOUT??

Bleeding……it's a normal thing in a woman's life, right? Something that we have come to live with for many years, most of us. Something that is a way of life, so we do not give it much of a second guess normally, right? But, what happens when the bleeding is not a normal thing? What happens when it is a signal to something much more serious going on in our bodies?

We live in a very fast paced world, and most often we women are very busy with our families, our work, and the many other obligations we have day to day. It is easy for us to not take the time to go and see a doctor, to brush things off as no big deal and worry about the other things going on in our lives. But the point of this book is that sometimes abnormal bleeding *is* a big deal. Sometimes our bodies may be telling us that there is a more serious problem going on. The hope is that if you see something in this book that is happening to you, then hopefully you will make an appointment with a doctor and get it checked out. Most times it may be no big deal, **but** there is always that one chance that it just **might** be a big deal.

This book was written with the hope that women who are having abnormal bleeding and/or spotting issues might take more notice and get themselves checked out with a doctor.

WHO AM I??

I am a wife, mother of 3, a grandmother and also a mom to 2 dogs (that number tends to fluctuate). I love animals, love to travel (when we can), love anything to do with the beach; snorkel, kayak and I learned how to scuba dive at the age of 50 (still learning, but it's a beautiful world underwater). As you can probably guess, I love the outdoors.

I have never written a book before now. This book was written completely on my research because of things that have happened to myself and other people I care about. I also am not a doctor, nor do I have any medical training whatsoever. So, none of this information is intended as medical advice (I will leave that to the medical professionals). These are just important facts that I have researched and believe every woman should be aware of. This book was written because a good friend of mine had similar problems to some of the things I talk about in this book. I also had my own scare at the age of 40. Because of these instances, it made me realize that a lot of women brush these symptoms off and do not get them checked out like we should. My friend may not have gotten treatment as soon if her sister hadn't had her own medical problem around the same time and insisted that she get checked by a doctor. So, my husband knew about all of this, kept persisting and asking me to write a book about it for other women. Since I am not a professional writer, I had no clue how to make this happen. But I started researching and writing and it started coming together. It is a simple little book, and my only hope with writing it is to get this information out to other women and make them aware.

Ch. 1 - Is this Menopause?? Or not??

She thought she was in menopause, she had not had a period for several months. So why was she now spotting blood? And more and more frequently? She thought it was probably normal, that her body was just adjusting to going through menopause. The spotting and bleeding continued off and on, but she may have continued to ignore it if it wasn't for the pressure of her sister to get herself examined.

This may be why so many women ignore the signs of abnormal bleeding problems. Not because we are naïve or clueless, but because we think that maybe the beginning stages of menopause may be causing this. We think that the occasional abnormal spotting or bleeding may just be our bodies way of adjusting. This is a very big change in our bodies, so we may not get too worried when we have some abnormal spotting or bleeding. And since we have been dealing with bleeding and/or spotting for most of our lives, we are not likely to get alarmed.

Maybe our periods have gotten more irregular, bleeding less, even skipping periods for a month or months at a time. So, we come to see this occasional bleeding as no big deal and not out of the ordinary. Maybe we are beginning to experience some other menopause signs besides our irregular periods, such as hot flashes, night sweats, mood swings, vaginal dryness, so we just assume that these times of bleeding are normal as our body gets used to this major change. Maybe we have put off having our regular pap smears for a while. Whether due to no medical insurance, money, time, or just the fact that we think since we are getting past child bearing age and entering menopause that it just isn't as important as it once was.

Well, this is what happened to a good friend of mine. She thought the abnormal bleeding and spotting was a normal thing for her body to be doing. She was in her early 50's and was experiencing some of the menopause symptoms I just mentioned. She figured it was no big deal, that she was just entering menopause. Besides, she was busy, and as many women do, we put things off because there are more important things to think about. Sometimes we lose track of how long it has been since we had a normal period maybe?

But that all changed when her sister had a uterine cancer scare and told her that she should also get checked out. It was then that my friend admitted what had been happening and got worried enough to visit the doctor. Thank goodness for that wake-up call, because when she did go in and get examined, she found out that she had what they believed at the time to be cancer.

Ch. 2 - My Own Story

I had my own cancer scare many years before that when I was only 40 years old. At that time, I was a working mother, had 3 children at home, my husband, dogs, cats, and life was busy. So, when I started spotting in between periods I brushed it off until it started becoming more and more frequent and the spotting was turning in to full blown bleeding in between periods. It got to the point that I was bleeding quite heavily a lot of the time. This definitely started to get my attention, probably because of the nuisance of constantly being worried about bleeding when I wasn't expecting it. I casually mentioned this to a friend I worked with one day, she said the same thing had happened to her around my age and it turned out that she had a fibroid tumor, which ended with her getting a hysterectomy.

So, I scheduled an appointment with a doctor and it turned out that yes, I did indeed have a uterine fibroid tumor. It was quite large by the time I went in and so we decided that since I would not be having any more children, it was in my best interest to just remove the tumor and the doctor would perform a partial hysterectomy at the same time. This was the action that myself, my husband and my doctor agreed upon. They tested the tumor and it was non-cancerous, which was a big relief. Come to find out that most uterine fibroid tumors are benign (non-cancerous), but at the time it was scary and I was worried until I received the news.

Now, I was not in menopause or even pre-menopause at the time that this happened to me, so even though this book was written geared more toward women near menopause, it can benefit any woman of any age. These things can happen to women of any age, so abnormal bleeding should always be checked out by your doctor.

Ch. 3 - Most Common Causes of Bleeding/Spotting

There are many different reasons that can cause abnormal bleeding, so I will list and go over some of the more common causes. But in any case, whether you are post menopause, just starting menopause, or even nowhere near menopause when you have abnormal bleeding, you should talk with your doctor. Regular pap smears and/or pelvic exams are a must! When caught early most of these problems can be taken care of, whereas if we let them go, sometimes the damage could be major.

 Some **(not all)** Causes of Abnormal Bleeding

- Uterine cancer
- Cervical cancer
- Cancer of the vagina
- Thinning/thickening of the tissues lining the uterus or vagina
- Uterine fibroids
- Polyps
- Medications
- Sexually transmitted diseases

In the following chapters, I will go over a brief description of some of these causes, symptoms and some of the treatments for them. While it is **_not_** a complete list of what may be wrong, it will give you an idea of the most common causes.

Ch. 4 - Uterine Cancer

Uterine cancer is cancer that forms in the tissues of the uterus. The growth of blood vessels that support cancer can result in vaginal bleeding. Bleeding is the most common symptom of Uterine Cancer *after* menopause. Bleeding can also sometimes be a sign of Cervical Cancer or Vaginal Cancer (see those chapters). The good news is that since uterine cancer is usually diagnosed in its early stages (usually when a woman experiences abnormal bleeding), there is a high cure rate.

<u>Symptoms of Uterine Cancer</u>

- Increasingly Heavy Periods
- Bleeding Between Periods
- Bleeding After Menopause

While a lot of times abnormal bleeding is *not* necessarily an indication of uterine cancer, **DO NOT** put off that trip to your doctor … and **DO NOT** wait for the bleeding to stop! Not only is the bleeding a nuisance, it could be a serious problem that you need to know about and take care of.

Ch. 5 - Cervical Cancer

Cervical cancer usually does not show any symptoms until the cancer has spread to other parts of the body, which is why it's so important to schedule routine Pap tests in addition to getting your *human papillomavirus* (HPV) vaccination. Once cervical cancer is more advanced, women may start to notice the following symptoms:

- Bleeding between menstrual periods
- Heavier menstrual periods
- Longer menstrual periods
- Bleeding after sexual intercourse
- Bleeding after menopause
- Bleeding after a pelvic exam

There are **other** symptoms of Cervical Cancer that you should be aware of besides abnormal vaginal bleeding; these are:

- Vaginal Discharge
- Pain during sexual intercourse
- Pelvic pain

- Leg pain or swelling
- Unexplained Weight Loss

Depending on the stage of cervical cancer, and if the cancer has spread, different types of treatment are used. Treatment is very effective if caught in the early stages, all the more reason why women need to be vigilant about getting pap smears and/or pelvic exams done regularly.

Standard methods of treatment typically used to treat cervical cancer are:

- Surgery
- Radiation therapy
- Chemotherapy
- Targeted therapy

Fortunately, the death rate from cervical cancer has decreased due to increased use of the pap smears and/or pelvic exams and also HPV vaccinations. It is important to understand how the HPV vaccine, regular exams and knowing the symptoms and warning signs of cervical cancer could save your life.

The ***most common cause of cervical cancer*** is human papillomavirus **(HPV)**, which is why getting all three doses of the *HPV vaccine* is important for both males and females. The CDC (Center for Disease Control) recommends:

- All children (male and female) ages 11-12 should get the HPV vaccine.
- Children (male and female) are encouraged to get all 3 doses of the vaccine at a young age, prior to being exposed to HPV, to maximize the effectiveness.
- If teenagers or young adults have not received the vaccine when they are younger, women can still get vaccinated through the age of 26 and men through the age of 21.

Ch. 6 - Cancer of the Vagina

Vaginal cancer is a disease in which malignant cancer cells form in the vagina. Vaginal cancer is not common and when found in early stages, it can often be cured. There are two main types of vaginal cancer: *squamous cell carcinoma* and *adenocarcinoma*. Risk factors for vaginal cancer include being age 60 or older, being exposed to DES while in the mother's womb, human papillomavirus (HPV) infection, having a history of abnormal cells in the cervix, and cervical cancer. To diagnose vaginal cancer, a doctor may do a pelvic exam, pap smear, biopsy, or colposcopy (a medical diagnostic procedure to examine an illuminated, magnified view of the cervix and the tissues of the vagina and vulva).

Symptoms of Vaginal Cancer

- Bleeding or discharge not related to menstrual periods.
- Pain during sexual intercourse
- Pain in the pelvic area
- A lump in the vagina.

<u>Treatment for Vaginal Cancer</u>

- Surgery
- Radiation therapy
- Chemotherapy

The prognosis will depend on the stage of the cancer and whether it has spread, as well as the size of the **tumor**, the grade of tumor cells, where the cancer is within the vagina, whether there are symptoms, the patient's age, general health, and whether the cancer has just been diagnosed or has recurred.

Ch. 7 - Thinning/Thickening of the Uterine lining and Thinning of the Vaginal Tissue

- Low hormone levels after menopause can cause the tissue that lines your uterus to get too *thin*. This may trigger bleeding.
- After menopause, your vaginal walls can become thin, dry and inflamed. This can lead to pain during sexual intercourse and also to bleeding, primarily after sex.
- Sometimes after menopause, the tissue that lines your uterus gets *thicker* and can bleed. If the cells become abnormal, this could lead to cancer.

Ch. 8 - Uterine Fibroids

Uterine fibroids are benign masses that grow in the uterus for unclear reasons. Uterine fibroids are commonly called by the shorter name, "fibroids". The medical term for a fibroid is leiomyoma, which refers to a proliferation or abnormal growth of smooth muscle tissue. They are usually not cancerous. Uterine fibroids can cause bleeding. This bleeding can sometimes be significant and lead to anemia. Fibroids are diagnosed by performing a manual pelvic examination and confirmed by ultrasound. In my case, I had an ultrasound done as well as an internal ultrasound to determine the size of the tumor.

Some of the reasons for surgical removal of uterine fibroids include:

1. If there is still concern that the uterine growth could be cancer. In these cases, the doctor is not certain that the growth is actually a benign fibroid. Unusually rapid growth is a sign that a uterine growth may be cancerous. The growth must be

removed and examined by a pathologist for signs of more dangerous conditions.
2. If another pelvic surgery is already being done (there are other reasons for pelvic surgery, such as ovarian disease).
3. If other medical treatments have failed to stop bleeding or other complications.

Most Common Types of Surgery for Fibroids

1. Hysterectomy: Removal of the uterus is called a hysterectomy. Fibroids are the most common reason that hysterectomies are performed in the United States. Advantages are that: (a) the fibroids never return (this is really the only "cure" for fibroids); (b) the woman will never have another menstrual period (which some, but not all women, find to be an advantage); and (c) contraception is no longer a concern. It is easy to understand, therefore, that the best candidates for a hysterectomy are not planning on having children in the future.
2. Myomectomy (Local Resection): This surgery involves the removal of the

fibroids themselves without removal of the whole uterus. Myomectomy is not permanent in the sense that fibroids can grow back after the procedure. The fibroids grow back in about 25% to 50% of women, and about 10% of women will need a second surgery. Although myomectomy is a sure temporary measure, it is less guaranteed to be a permanent solution. Thus, this procedure is often used to "buy time" if the woman is planning to become pregnant in the next few years. The advantages of this surgery are that it preserves the uterus for childbearing and involves less extensive surgery, which results in less extensive recovery periods. Following this surgery bleeding tends to be much improved after (in about 80% of women). This is a valuable option if the woman is still planning to have children or unsure if she will want to have children in the future.

3. Embolization: Another technique for treating fibroids is known as uterine artery embolization (UAE). This technique uses small beads of a compound called

polyvinyl alcohol, which is injected through a catheter into the arteries that supply the fibroid. These beads obstruct the blood supply to the fibroid and starve it of blood and oxygen. Uterine artery occlusion (UAO), which involves clamping the involved uterine arteries as opposed to injecting the polyvinyl alcohol beads, has also been used to interrupt blood supply to the fibroid.

There are some other procedures such as boring holes into the fibroid with laser fibers, freezing probes (cryosurgery), and other destructive techniques that do not actually remove the tissue but try to destroy it in place. These are the most common surgeries and treatments that are used by doctors to treat uterine fibroids. If you have this problem, you will need to talk with your doctor and find the best option for yourself.

Ch. 9 – Polyps

These tissue growths show up inside your uterus or cervical canal, or on your cervix. They are usually not cancer, but they can cause spotting, heavy bleeding, and/or bleeding after sex. Sometimes polyps cause such light spotting you barely even need a pad, or they can cause heavier flows, especially if they get larger. Cervical polyps can also cause increased discharge. It may be a white or yellow mucus. It can also seem like just more than usual amounts of your normal discharge, so it's not necessarily an obvious (or particularly troublesome) symptom.

The treatment varies depending upon if the polyps are giving you problems or if the polyp appears atypical. If you are experiencing symptoms, the treatment is generally just to remove the polyp. It is usually a simple in-office procedure, sometimes involving anesthesia, but often not. After removal, polyps do not usually grow back, but new ones can pop up.
The treatment if your polyp(s) appear atypical (even if you don't have symptoms) is usually to

play it safe and remove it. Polyps have a particular look to them, according to medical professionals, so if the polyp looks odd, those are the times a doctor might worry. If there's any chance the growth could be cancerous, doctors will usually play it safe and want to remove it.

Ch. 10 – Medications

Sometimes medications that we are taking can have some strange side effects. Abnormal bleeding can often be a side effect of some drugs such as hormone therapy, tamoxifen or blood thinners. If you are taking these medications or others and begin having abnormal bleeding, talk to your doctor to determine the cause.

Ch. 11 - Sexually Transmitted Diseases

Another cause of abnormal bleeding is something many of us might not think about. Some STDs such as chlamydia and gonorrhea may cause spotting and/or bleeding after sex. Genital herpes sores may also bleed. If you know you have an STD and experience abnormal bleeding, you should get checked out by a doctor to rule out any other problems. If you are not aware of any STD but are experiencing abnormal bleeding, get checked out by a doctor to determine the cause.

Pap Smear Guidelines

According to the CDC (Centers for Disease Control and Prevention), they recommend women get their Pap test done from ages 21 to 65 years old. The pap test, which screens for cervical cancer, is one of the most reliable and effective cancer screening tests available. doctors will have different suggestions for how often you need to have your Pap test done, usually every 2-3 years while you are younger, sometimes longer in between as you get older; barring any symptoms, risk factors, past Pap tests that were abnormal or a family history. If you are older and have had normal Pap test results for many years, or have had your cervix removed during a total hysterectomy, your doctor may tell you that you do not need a Pap test as often, or maybe not at all. But let the doctor advise you on that, do not make that decision on your own.

If you are 30 years old or older, you may choose to have an HPV test along with your Pap test. Both tests can be performed by your doctor at the same time. When you have both tests performed together, this is called *co-testing.* If your test results are normal, your chance of getting cervical cancer in the next few years is very low. You may then be able to wait as long as 5 years before your next screening, but you should still get regular checkups.

Even if you have a Pap smear done regularly and they have been normal if you notice signs or symptoms that are unusual, see your doctor to find out what is happening.

CONCLUSION

Now as far as what happened to my friend I mentioned earlier who had the cancer scare. Once she went to the doctor, things moved quickly. She had surgery within a couple of days; the tumor was removed, tested and determined non-cancerous. I do know that her doctor said it was a very good thing that she came in when she did. She was very relieved and of course, glad that her sister had pushed her to get that examination. They were both in their very early 50's at the time this happened to each of them.

After talking about this and hearing my friend say that she wasn't really worried about it until her sister called her, I know that a lot of women are like this. As we talked more about it, my husband kept telling me that other women need to know this and gently pressured me until I wrote this book. And he is right! We don't always get worried until things get more severe, and we may not realize that something like this could be such a big thing. Women do need to be made aware of this and get regular checkups with their doctors. If this book can help raise awareness to at least one person, then it is more than worth it to me. Please pay attention to your bodies and if something seems abnormal, then get to your doctor and get checked out. And please feel free to share this information with friends or family that may benefit from this information.

I thank you for taking the time to read this and I hope that you were able to get some useful information out of it.